Blood Type Diet

A Comprehensive Step-by-Step Guide to Optimizing Your Health and Well-Being Based on Your Blood Type

By Travis R. Burkhart

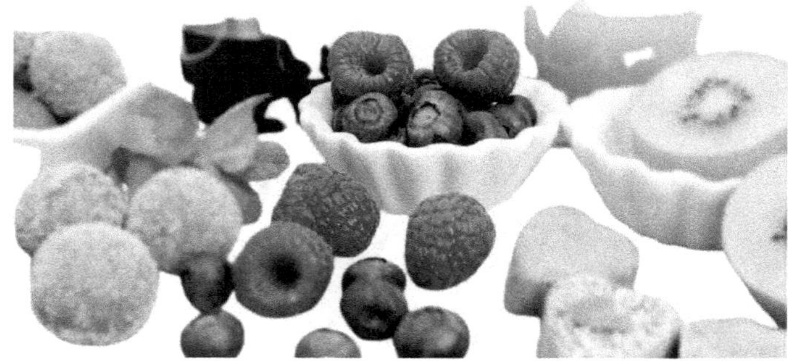

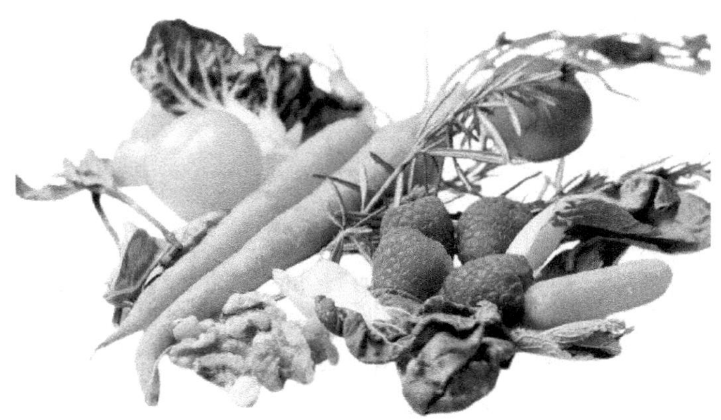

INTRODUCTION

Welcome to a voyage of self-discovery and optimum health made possible by the Blood Type Diet's revolutionary power. This ground-breaking book takes us on an exploration of the complex relationships that exist between our blood types and the foods we eat, providing us with a deep new understanding of how our bodies function best when fed by their genetic blueprints.

Suppose you could figure out the key to your body's most energetic state of being, one in which energy is abundant, controlling your weight becomes simple, and vitality is radiated from the inside. Your body's potential may be fully realized with the help of the Blood Type Diet, which can lead you toward a customized nutrition plan that goes beyond fads and trends.

Get ready to go on a journey of empowerment, change, and discovery as we dig into the pages of this book. We'll explore the different dietary recommendations for blood types O, A, B, and AB as we work together to solve the puzzles around blood type research. Each chapter uncovers the specific nutritional blueprint that corresponds with your genetic ancestry, from the plant-based preferences of blood type A to the ancestral knowledge of blood type O for blood types.

The Blood Type Diet, however, is a comprehensive approach to well-being that takes into account one's mind, body, and spirit rather than just a set of food guidelines. You'll discover how to nurture every part of your being and create a life of bright health and vitality with helpful advice on exercise, stress reduction, and sleep optimization.

Are you prepared to set out on a path to become the happiest, healthiest version of yourself? Come along with me as we explore the Blood Type Diet's possibilities and embrace a way of life that values our uniqueness. Together, let's set out on this life-changing adventure and uncover the radiant well-being that lies inside.

CHAPTER 1

Understanding the Blood Type Diet

Welcome to the start of your adventure using the Blood Type Diet to achieve maximum health and well-being. We'll explore the core ideas of this ground-breaking approach to wellness and nutrition in this chapter. By the conclusion, you'll know exactly how your blood type affects what you need to eat and how to use that information to reach your health objectives.

First Step: Overview of the Blood Type Diet

Start by becoming familiar with the fundamental ideas behind the Blood Type Diet. Be aware that the foundation of this diet is the theory that your blood type influences how your body responds to different meals.

Recognize that every blood type (O, A, B, and AB) has distinct traits and inclinations, such as variations in immune system performance, digestive enzyme levels, and general health vulnerabilities.

Stress that the Blood Type Diet is a customized dietary plan based on a person's blood type rather than a one-size-fits-all approach to nutrition.

Step 2: Examining Blood Type Features

Find out about the characteristics that set each blood type apart. People with blood type O, for instance, are sometimes referred to as "hunters" who thrive on animal protein, whereas people with blood type A are thought to be better off eating a plant-based diet.

Recognize the importance of blood type antigens and how they affect the body's reactions to different meals, environments, and stressors.

Consider your blood type and how it corresponds with the traits and dietary guidelines that go along with it.

Step 3: The Science Behind the Blood Type Diet

Delve into the scientific research and theories that underpin the Blood Type Diet. Explore studies that have examined the relationship between blood type and susceptibility to certain diseases, as well as the impact of blood type on nutrient metabolism and immune function.

Consider the evolutionary perspective of the Blood Type Diet, which posits that each blood type evolved in response to specific dietary and environmental factors over thousands of years.

Appreciate the holistic approach of the Blood Type Diet, which considers not only the nutritional aspects but also the psychological and emotional factors that influence health and well-being.

Step 4: Benefits of the Blood Type Diet

Explore the potential benefits of following the Blood Type Diet, including improved digestion, enhanced immune function, increased energy levels, and weight management.

Understand that the personalized nature of the Blood Type Diet allows for targeted interventions to address individual health concerns and optimize overall wellness.

Hear success stories from individuals who have experienced transformative changes in their health and quality of life through adherence to the Blood Type Diet.

Step 5: Getting Started

Take the first steps toward incorporating the principles of the Blood Type Diet into your lifestyle. Begin by identifying your blood type through a simple blood test or by consulting your healthcare provider.

Set realistic goals and expectations for your journey with the Blood Type Diet. Understand that change takes time and commitment, but the potential benefits are well worth the effort.

Stay open-minded and curious as you embark on this journey of self-discovery and transformation through the power of personalized nutrition.

Congratulations on completing Chapter 1! You are now equipped with the foundational knowledge needed to embark on your blood-type diet journey. In the chapters to come, we will delve deeper into each blood type and provide practical guidance on how to optimize your health and well-being based on your unique biological blueprint.

CHAPTER 2

Blood Type O Diet Plan

Welcome to Chapter 2 of your Blood Type Diet journey, tailored specifically for individuals with blood type O. In this chapter, we will provide you with a detailed and comprehensive diet plan designed to optimize your health and well-being based on your unique blood type characteristics. Follow these step-by-step guidelines to discover the foods that support your body's needs and thrive on the Blood Type O Diet.

Step 1: Understanding Blood Type O Characteristics

Review the key characteristics associated with blood type O, such as the ancestral "hunter" archetype and the strong digestive system optimized for animal protein consumption.

Acknowledge the tendency for individuals with blood type O to thrive on high-protein, low-carbohydrate diets and to excel in activities that require strength and endurance.

Reflect on how these characteristics align with your own experiences and preferences, setting the stage for personalized dietary recommendations.

Step 2: Beneficial Foods for Blood Type O

Identify the foods that are most beneficial for individuals with blood type O. These include lean meats such as beef, lamb, and venison, as well as seafood such as salmon, mackerel, and cod.

Emphasize the importance of incorporating plenty of fresh fruits and vegetables into your diet, with an emphasis on leafy greens, cruciferous vegetables, and berries.

Discuss the benefits of consuming moderate amounts of healthy fats from sources such as olive oil, avocado, and nuts, which provide essential nutrients and support overall health.

Step 3: items to Minimize or Avoid

List the items that people with blood type O should limit or stay away from to maintain optimal health. These include cereals like wheat and corn, which can induce inflammation, and dairy products, which can be difficult to digest.

Talk about the possible adverse effects of beans and legumes on those with blood type O because of their lectin content and ability to cause digestive problems.

Promote cutting back on or giving up processed and refined foods, as well as artificial sweeteners and additives, as these can exacerbate health problems and counteract the advantages of the Blood Type O Diet.

Step 4: Blood Type O Meal Plans Example

Offer sample menus that show you how to arrange your meals according to the Blood Type O Diet's tenets. To guarantee balanced nutrition and satisfaction, include a range of nutrient-dense foods.

Serve Blood Type O-friendly foods for breakfast, lunch, supper, and snacks that highlight their flavor and adaptability, like turkey lettuce wraps, grilled salmon with steamed broccoli, and omelets with veggies.

To keep meals engaging and pleasurable while still following the Blood Type O Diet's recommendations, experiment with flavors and ingredients.

Step 5: Useful Advice for Success

Provide helpful advice to people with blood type O so they can successfully follow the diet plan in their everyday lives. These could include techniques for organizing and preparing meals, advice on grocery shopping, and rules for dining out.

Promote mindful eating techniques, such as observing how different foods make you feel and paying attention to indications about hunger and fullness.

Stress the value of endurance, adaptability, and consistency as you traverse the opportunities and challenges of adhering to the Blood Type O Diet.

Congratulations on completing Chapter 2! By following these step-by-step guidelines and personalized recommendations, you are well on your way to harnessing the power of the Blood Type O Diet to optimize your health and well-being. In the chapters to come, we will continue to explore the unique dietary needs and preferences of each blood type, empowering you to make informed choices and achieve lasting results.

CHAPTER 3

Blood Type A Diet Plan

Designed especially for those with blood type A, welcome to Chapter 3 of your Blood Type Diet journey. We will present you with a thorough food plan in this chapter that is tailored to your specific blood type to maximize health and well-being. Discover the foods that complement your body's demands and flourish on the Blood Type A Diet by following these easy-to-follow steps.

Step 1: Recognizing the Features of Blood Type A

Go over the main traits of blood type A, including the ancestor "cultivator" archetype and the propensity for a diet high in plants.

Recognize the possibility that people with blood type A may be sensitive to specific foods, including dairy and animal proteins.

To provide individualized nutritional recommendations, consider how these traits fit with your own experiences and preferences.

Step 2: Beneficial Foods for Blood Type A

Identify the foods that are most beneficial for individuals with blood type A. These include a variety of fresh fruits and vegetables, with an emphasis on plant-based proteins such as legumes, tofu, and tempeh.

Discuss the benefits of consuming whole grains such as quinoa, brown rice, and oats, which provide essential nutrients and fiber while supporting digestive health.

Highlight the importance of incorporating fermented foods like miso, kimchi, and sauerkraut, which can support gut health and immune function.

Step 3: Foods to Reduce or Steer Clear off

Emphasize the foods that people with blood type A should limit or stay away from to maintain optimal health. Red meat is one of them since it can be hard to digest and cause inflammation.

Talk about the possible adverse effects of dairy products on people with blood type A, including the possibility of immunological reactions and lactose intolerance.

Promote cutting back on or giving up processed and refined meals, alcohol, and caffeine, which can throw off hormone balance and energy levels.

Step 4: Blood Type A Meal Plan Samples

Give examples of meal plans that show you how to arrange your meals according to the Blood Type A Diet's tenets. Incorporate a range of plant-based foods to guarantee well-balanced nourishment and contentment.

Serve Blood Type A-friendly dishes for breakfast, lunch, supper, and snacks that highlight their flavor and adaptability, like quinoa salad with mixed vegetables, lentil soup with whole grain bread, and vegetable stir-fry with tofu.

While following the Blood Type A Diet's guidelines, encourage creativity and experimentation with flavors and ingredients to make meals interesting and pleasurable.

Step 5: Useful Advice for Success

Provide useful advice to help people with blood type A effectively follow the food plan daily. These could include techniques for organizing and preparing meals, advice on grocery shopping, and rules for dining out.

Promote mindful eating techniques, such as chewing carefully, enjoying every meal, and observing your emotional response to various foods. Stress the value of paying attention to your body's cues and modifying the blood type A diet as necessary to maintain your health and well-being.

Congratulations on completing Chapter 3! By following these step-by-step guidelines and personalized recommendations, you are well on your way to harnessing the power of the Blood Type A Diet to optimize your health and well-being. In the chapters to come, we will continue to explore the unique dietary needs and preferences of each blood type, empowering you to make informed choices and achieve lasting results.

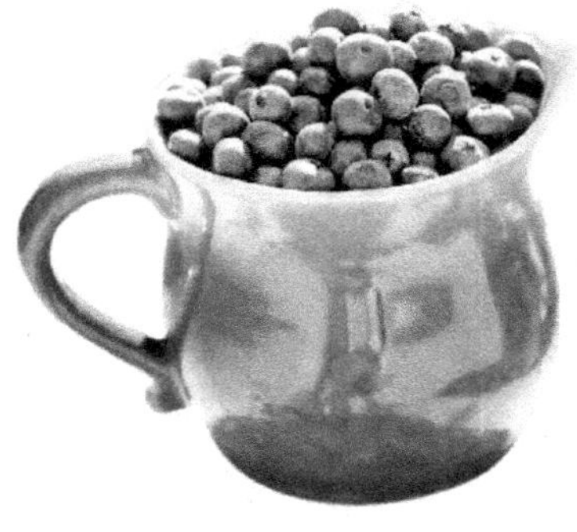

CHAPTER 4

Blood Type B Diet Plan

Designed especially for those with blood type B, welcome to Chapter 4 of your Blood Type Diet journey. We will present you with a thorough food plan in this chapter that is tailored to your specific blood type to maximize health and well-being. Discover the foods that meet your body's demands and flourish on the Blood Type B Diet by following these simple instructions.

Step 1: Recognizing the Features of Blood Type B

Go over the main traits of blood type B, including the ancestry of the "nomad" archetype and the capacity to live on a variety of foods.

Recognize the adaptability and flexibility of people with blood type B, who could benefit from a balance of various food categories and cooking styles.

Consider how these traits coincide with your own experiences and tastes, laying the groundwork for customized food suggestions.

Step 2: Blood Type B-Friendly Foods

Determine which foods are most healthy for people with blood type B. These comprise a wide variety of meals, including dairy items like yogurt and cheese and lean meats like lamb, turkey, and fish.

Talk about the advantages of eating a range of fruits and vegetables, with a focus on cruciferous vegetables, leafy greens, and berries.

Emphasize the value of eating whole grains, which improve digestive health and offer vital nutrients.

Examples of such grains are rice, oats, and buckwheat.

Step 3: items to Minimize or Avoid

List the items that people with blood type B should limit or stay away from to maintain optimal health. These could include meats that are less suitable for blood type B digestion, such as pork and chicken.

Talk about the possible lectin reactions and digestive problems that wheat and corn may cause in people with blood type B

.

Step 4: Sample Meal Plans for Blood Type B

Promote cutting back on or giving up processed and refined meals, alcohol, and caffeine, which can throw off hormone balance and energy levels.

Give examples of meal plans that show you how to arrange your meals according to the Blood Type B Diet's tenets. Incorporate a range of foods from various food groups to guarantee well-rounded nourishment and contentment.

Serve Blood Type B-friendly foods for breakfast, lunch, supper, and snacks that highlight their flavor and adaptability, like grilled salmon with quinoa salad, turkey and avocado wraps, and stir-fried vegetables with tofu.

To keep meals engaging and pleasurable while still following the Blood Type B Diet's requirements, experiment with flavors and cuisines.

Step 5: Useful Advice for Success

Provide helpful advice to people with blood type B so they may successfully follow the diet plan daily. These could include techniques for organizing and preparing meals, advice on grocery shopping, and rules for dining out.

Promote mindful eating techniques, such as observing signs of hunger and fullness and observing the emotional impact of certain foods. Stress the value of keeping a varied and balanced diet while also respecting the special dietary requirements and preferences of people with blood type B.

.

Congratulations on completing Chapter 4! By following these step-by-step guidelines and personalized recommendations, you are well on your way to harnessing the power of the Blood Type B Diet to optimize your health and well-being. In the chapters to come, we will continue to explore the unique dietary needs and preferences of each blood type, empowering you to make informed choices and achieve lasting results.

CHAPTER 5

Blood Type AB Diet Plan

Especially for those with blood type AB, welcome to Chapter 5 of your blood type diet journey. We will present you with a thorough food plan in this chapter that is tailored to your specific blood type to maximize health and well-being. Discover the foods that complement your body's needs and flourish on the Blood Type AB Diet by following these easy-to-follow steps.

Step 1: Recognizing the Features of Blood Type AB

Go over the essential features of blood type AB, which blends features from blood types A and B. People who have blood type AB are frequently described as possessing a special combination of sensitivity and adaptability.

Recognize that people with blood type AB must strike a balance between the A and B blood type requirements, combining aspects of both plant-based and omnivorous diets.

Consider how these traits coincide with your own experiences and food preferences to create customized dietary suggestions.

.

Step 2: Blood Type AB-Friendly Foods

Determine which foods are best for people with blood type AB. These comprise an extensive range of meals, including dairy products, seafood, tofu, and a colorful assortment of fruits and vegetables.

Talk about the advantages of including both plant-based proteins, such as beans, and legumes, and lean proteins, like fish and turkey, in your diet.

Stress the value of eating whole grains, which include quinoa, rice, and oats, to supply vital nutrients and improve digestive health.

Step 3: items to Minimize or Avoid

List the items that people with blood type AB should limit or stay away from to maintain optimal health. These could include meats like pork and beef, which might not be as well suited for blood-type AB digestion.

Talk about the possible adverse effects of gluten-containing grains and dairy products for blood type AB individuals, including the possibility of immunological reactions and digestive problems.

Promote cutting back on or giving up processed and refined meals, alcohol, and caffeine, which can adversely affect one's energy and general well-being.

Step 4: Sample Meal Plans for Blood Type AB

Provide sample meal plans that demonstrate how to arrange your meals in line with the principles of the Blood Type AB Diet. Include a variety of meals from different food groups to provide a well-rounded diet and satisfaction.

For breakfast, lunch, dinner, and snacks, serve Blood Type AB-friendly dishes that emphasize their flavor and versatility, such as lentil soup with whole grain bread, avocado and salmon salad, and stir-fried veggies and tofu.

Try different flavors and cuisines to make meals interesting and enjoyable while adhering to the Blood Type AB Diet guidelines.

Step 5: Practical Tips for Success

Provide helpful advice on how people with blood type AB can successfully incorporate the diet plan into their everyday lives. These could include techniques for organizing and preparing meals, advice on grocery shopping, and rules for dining out.

Promote mindful eating techniques, such as observing your body's signals of hunger and fullness and observing the emotional impact of various foods.

Stress the value of developing a customized strategy that supports your health and well-being on the Blood Type AB Diet by combining components from both blood types A and B.

Congratulations on completing Chapter 5! By following these step-by-step guidelines and personalized recommendations, you are well on your way to harnessing the power of the Blood Type AB Diet to optimize your health and well-being. In the chapters to come, we will continue to explore the unique dietary needs and preferences of each blood type, empowering you to make informed choices and achieve lasting results.

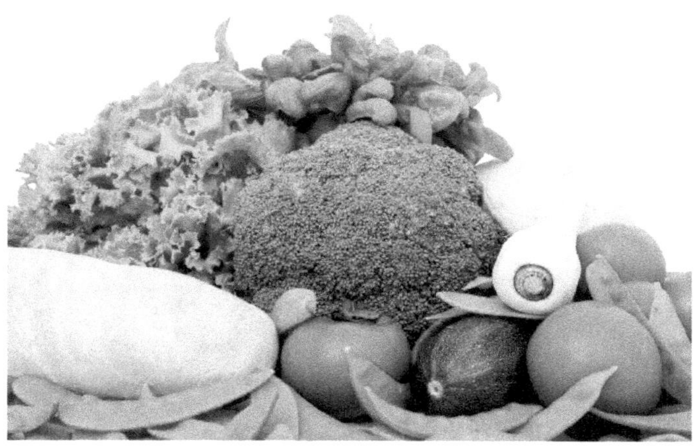

CHAPTER 6

Shopping for Success

Welcome to your sixth chapter on the Blood Type Diet! We'll look at the key elements of successful blood type-specific grocery shopping in this chapter. You'll discover how to organize the proper supplies in your pantry and make wise decisions when shopping the store aisles by adhering to these detailed instructions.

Step 1: Recognizing the Dietary Requirements for Your Blood Type

Start by going over the dietary guidelines described in earlier chapters that are particular to your blood type (O, A, B, or AB). Recognize the kinds of meals that are best for your blood type and which ones you should limit or avoid.

Remember any allergies or food sensitivities you may have, along with any particular health objectives you hope to accomplish with your diet.

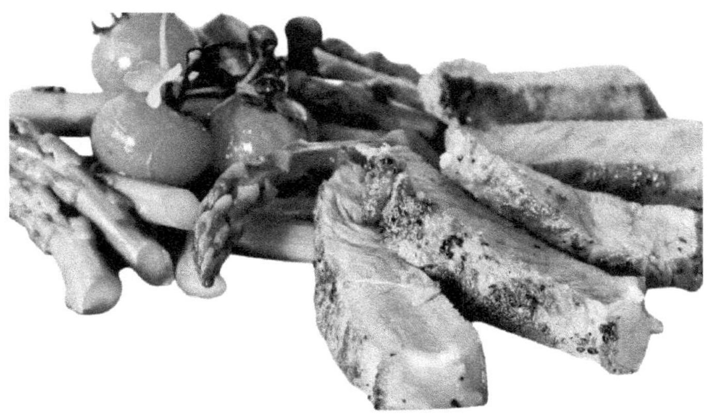

Step 2: Make a Shopping List

Spend some time making a thorough shopping list based on your blood type diet, meal planning, and suggestions before you go to the grocery store. To guarantee a balanced diet, incorporate a range of foods from various dietary categories.

List goods according to grocery store departments (fruit, dairy, meats, etc.) to make your trip to the store easier and prevent you from forgetting anything.

Step 3: Select Fresh, Whole Foods

Whenever possible, choose seasonal, fresh produce when choosing fruits and vegetables. To make sure you're getting a wide spectrum of nutrients, choose a diversity of hues. Look in the bulk or whole foods department for whole grains, including oats, brown rice, and quinoa. Steer clear of refined and processed grains, as they might not be as good for your blood type.

Step 4: Choose Lean Proteins

Make sure the sources of lean protein you choose match the guidelines for your blood type. Lean meats like beef and chicken are ideal for blood type O people, while tofu and lentils are good sources of plant-based protein for blood type A people.

Choose premium, sustainably sourced fish, such as mackerel and salmon, which are rich in protein and necessary omega-3 fatty acids.

Step 5: Carefully Read Food Labels

Spend some time reading food labels to find any components that may not be good for your blood type. Steer clear of goods that include artificial flavors or sweeteners, preservatives, or additives.

Make sure the products you select fit your dietary requirements and tastes by paying attention to ingredient lists and allergen warnings.

Step 6: Fill Your Pantry with Blood Type-Friendly Staples

Make sure to fill your pantry with items that are appropriate for your blood type and those you'll use frequently in your meals. Olive oil, herbs and spices, nuts and seeds, and whole grain flavoring are a few examples of this.

Think about stocking up on a range of sauces and condiments that go well with your blood type. For example, blood types A and B should use balsamic vinegar and tamari sauce, respectively.

Step 7: Stay Hydrated

Don't forget to put water on your list of things to buy! Select hydrating liquids such as herbal teas, water, and others based on your blood type.

Avoid or limit sugar-filled beverages, such as sodas, as they can aggravate inflammation and cause other health problems.

.

Step 8: Plan for Success

Lastly, schedule your shopping excursion during a time when you'll be relaxed and well-rested, allowing you to concentrate on making well-considered decisions. If you're looking for unusual, fresh products, try visiting your neighborhood farmers' markets or specialized shops. After your shopping excursion, spend some time arranging your groceries and supplies for meal prep so you can quickly find them when it's time to cook.

If you adhere to these detailed tips for successful shopping, you'll be prepared to stock your kitchen with the appropriate foods to support your blood type diet. We'll look at meal preparation and planning techniques in the upcoming chapter to help you make the most of those ingredients and eat tasty, nutrient-dense meals catered to your dietary requirements.

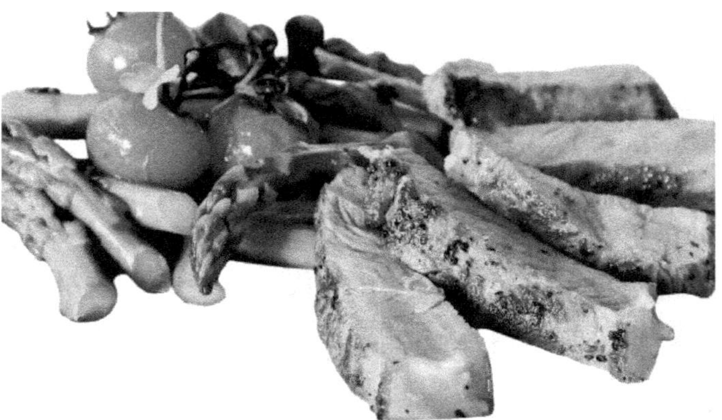

CHAPTER 7

Meal Preparation and Planning

Welcome to your seventh chapter on the Blood Type Diet! In this chapter, we will explore the crucial procedures for meal planning and preparation specific to your blood type. You'll discover how to quickly plan and cook wholesome meals that fit your dietary requirements by following these step-by-step instructions, making it simpler to stick to your health objectives.

Step1: Examine the Dietary Guidelines for Your Blood Type

Start by going over the food suggestions that are particular to your blood type that were covered in previous chapters. Make a list of foods that are good for your blood type and those that you should limit or stay away from.

Make sure you're including the correct ratio of nutrients in your meals to meet your body's requirements by basing your meal planning decisions on this knowledge.

Step 2: Schedule Meal Planning Time

Set aside time every week to prepare your meals for the next few days. You can choose any time that is most convenient for you for this, even a weekend afternoon.

Considering your daily activities and schedule, make a meal planning schedule that includes breakfast, lunch, dinner, and snacks.

Step 3: Make a menu and select recipes

Make recipe choices based on dietary rules and preferences specific to your blood type. Seek ideas from cookbooks, the internet, or well-received recipes from the past.

To keep things fresh, create a weekly menu with a range of meals and snacks that feature several food categories and flavors.

Step 4: Create a Shopping List

Create a detailed shopping list that includes all the ingredients you'll need for the week based on your menu and recipes. To make your grocery shopping trip go more smoothly, divide your list into regions of the supermarket.

To help you avoid making unnecessary purchases, verify whether any of the goods on your list are already in your pantry or refrigerator.

.

Step 5: Prepare Ingredients Ahead of Time

To increase the efficiency of cooking over the week, schedule time for ingredient prep. This could be pre-cooking grains and legumes, cleaning and cutting veggies, or marinating proteins.

To keep prepared goods fresh until you're ready to use them, store them in the refrigerator in airtight containers or resealable bags.

Step 6: Batch Cook Whenever Possible

To have meals ready to go throughout the week, think about batch cooking greater quantities of particular recipes or ingredients. This might apply to grains, casseroles, stews, and soups.

To make quick grab-and-go dinners on hectic days, divide up batch-cooked meals into individual servings and keep them in the freezer or refrigerator.

Step 7: Include Flexibility and Variety

To make your meals engaging and pleasurable, try to include a range of tastes, textures, and cuisines in your meal preparation. Try out different ingredients and dishes without fear. Stay adaptable and ready to make changes when necessary, particularly if your plans alter or unforeseen circumstances arise throughout the workweek.

Step 8: Pay Attention to Your Body and Watch Portion Sizes

During meals, be mindful of portion sizes and attentive to your body's signals of hunger and fullness. Aim for well-balanced, filling meals rather than binge eating or restricting yourself.

To assist manage portion sizes, think about using smaller plates or bowls. You can also practice mindful eating by chewing deeply and appreciating each bite.

.

By following these step-by-step guidelines for meal preparation and planning, you'll be better equipped to incorporate the principles of the Blood Type Diet into your daily routine. In the next chapter, we'll explore strategies for dining out while staying true to your blood type dietary recommendations, ensuring that you can enjoy meals both at home and away from home while supporting your health and well-being.

CHAPTER 8

Eating Out on the Blood Type Diet

Welcome to your eighth chapter on the Blood Type Diet! This chapter will discuss doable tactics for eating out that nevertheless adhere to blood-type-specific dietary guidelines. You can eat outside of your home while maintaining your health and well-being by adhering to these detailed rules, which will teach you how to make wise decisions at restaurants and social events.

Step 1: Find Restaurants in Advance

Before going out to eat, spend some time finding local restaurants that have menu items that are appropriate for your blood type. Seek out restaurants that respect dietary restrictions and place an emphasis on using entire, fresh products.

Look through internet menus, reviews, and ratings to get a sense of what kinds of dishes are offered and how well they fit into your dietary requirements.

Step 2: Plan Your Order

After selecting a restaurant, go over the menu beforehand and make your order according to the nutritional guidelines for your blood type. Seek out recipes that include healthy grains, fresh veggies, and lean proteins.

To make sure your dietary requirements are met, think about getting in touch with the restaurant in advance to ask about possible ingredient changes or substitutes.

Step 3: Use the Menu Wisely

When you get to the restaurant, look over the menu carefully and, if necessary, ask your waitress for assistance. Make it clear what foods you enjoy to eat and any special dietary requirements you may have.

Look for menu options like vegetable stir-fries, salads with grilled chicken or seafood, or lean protein-based dishes that closely correspond to your blood type recommendations.

Step 4: Customize Your Order

Don't hesitate to alter your order to better accommodate any dietary requirements. Request steamed or mildly cooked vegetables, ask for dressings and sauces on the side, and, if available, choose whole grain or gluten-free alternatives.

Tell your waitress about any dietary restrictions or allergies to guarantee that your food is prepared properly and according to your requirements.

Step 5: Exercise Portion Control

When dining out, pay attention to the portion sizes you eat because restaurant dishes are sometimes larger than what you might eat at home. If an entree is served, think about splitting it with a dining partner or requesting a half quantity.

Throughout the meal, pay attention to your body's signals of hunger and fullness. Stop eating when you're satisfied, rather than when you're too full.

Step 6: Remain Hydrated

When dining out, don't forget to stay hydrated by consuming water or other non-alcoholic drinks. Restrict your use of alcoholic and sugary drinks, as they may contain more calories and not be suitable for your blood type.

It is advisable to have a reusable water bottle so that you can stay hydrated during your dinner.

Step 7: Savor the Experience

Lastly, don't forget to savor the occasion of going out to eat with friends or family. Pay attention to the fun of sharing a meal with others and experiencing different flavors and cultures. Aim for moderation and balance instead of perfection, and have faith that one meal won't unduly hinder your overall success on the Blood Type Diet.

By following these step-by-step guidelines for dining out on the Blood Type Diet, you'll be better equipped to make informed choices and enjoy meals outside of your home while supporting your health and well-being. In the next chapter, we'll explore strategies for managing stress and improving sleep, two essential components of overall wellness that can complement your dietary efforts.

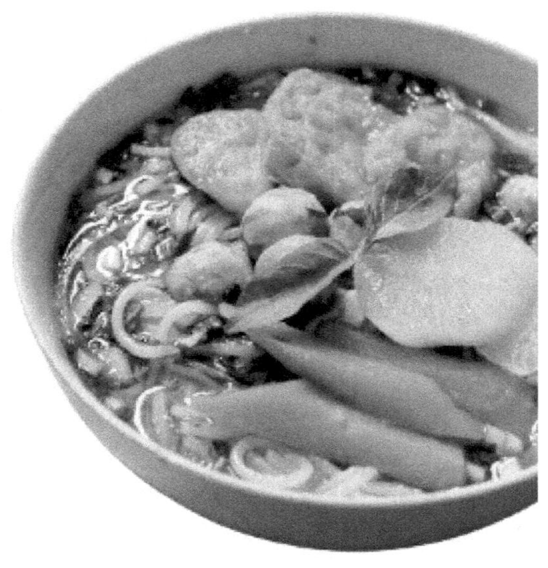

CHAPTER 9

Exercise and Lifestyle Recommendations

Welcome to your ninth chapter on the Blood Type Diet! This chapter will discuss the value of physical activity and lifestyle choices that enhance overall health and nutrition. You can optimize the benefits of the Blood Type Diet by learning how to include physical exercise and healthy lifestyle habits into your daily routine according to these detailed suggestions.

First, determine your present activity level.

Start by evaluating your existing lifestyle choices and degree of physical exercise. Think about the frequency of your activity, the kinds of things you want to do, and any obstacles or difficulties you could have in maintaining an active lifestyle.

Reflect on your daily routine and identify opportunities to incorporate more movement and physical exercise throughout the day, such as going for quick walks, taking the stairs rather than the elevator, or engaging in physically demanding hobbies.

Step 2: Set Achievable Activity Goals

Based on your present level of fitness, health, and personal preferences, set attainable activity goals. To enhance general health and well-being, try to incorporate aerobic activity with strength training, flexibility, and balancing exercises.

As your fitness increases, start with simple, manageable goals and progressively raise the frequency, duration, and intensity of your workouts.

Step 3: Select Pleasurable Activities

Pick out physical pursuits and workouts that you look forward to and like. Find activities that suit your lifestyle and something you enjoy, whether it's walking, jogging, cycling, swimming, dancing, yoga, or martial arts.

Try a variety of fitness routines to avoid getting bored and keep things fresh. To incorporate a social component into your workouts, think about signing up for sports leagues or group fitness courses.

.

Step 4: Make Exercise a Regular Part of Your Schedule

Plan regular workouts into your weekly schedule, just like you would any other significant event or obligation. Aim for at least 150 minutes per week, spaced out over many days, of moderate-intensity aerobic activity or 75 minutes of vigorous-intensity activity.

If necessary, divide up longer workout sessions into small bursts throughout the day. For example, take brisk 10-minute walks or perform fast bodyweight exercises while taking a break from work.

Step 5: Listen to Your Body and Rest

Pay attention to the cues your body gives you and modify the time and intensity of your workouts accordingly. Keep an eye out for any indications of exhaustion, pain, or discomfort, and allow yourself time to recuperate as necessary.

Include rest days in your weekly workout regimen to give your body a chance to rebuild and repair muscle. On your days off, spend time doing light exercises like yoga, stretching, or leisurely walks.

Step 6: Be Active All Throughout the Day

Seek chances to engage in physical activity outside of scheduled training sessions. Use the stairs rather than the elevator, go short distances by foot or bicycle rather than by car, and stand up or move around when engaging in sedentary activities like watching TV or working at a desk.

To help you remember to move throughout the day, set alarms or reminders. You can also use apps or activity trackers to keep track of your daily steps and your progress toward your objectives.

Step 7: Give Sleep and Stress Management Priority

Acknowledge the role that both stress management and restful sleep play in promoting general health and well-being. For maximum benefit, aim for 7-9 hours of sound sleep each night and stick to a regular sleep pattern.

To help control tension and encourage relaxation, try stress-reduction methods including progressive muscle relaxation, yoga, meditation, and deep breathing. Set aside time for the things that make you happy and fulfilled, and if you need help, ask friends, family, or mental health specialists for it.

By following these step-by-step guidelines for exercise and lifestyle recommendations, you'll be better equipped to incorporate physical activity and healthy habits into your daily routine, enhancing the benefits of the Blood Type Diet and supporting your overall health and well-being. In the next chapter, we'll explore strategies for managing stress and improving sleep, two essential components of overall wellness that can complement your dietary efforts.

CHAPTER 10

Managing Stress and Improving Sleep

Welcome to your Blood Type Diet journey's Chapter 10! This chapter will include helpful techniques for reducing stress and enhancing sleep, two aspects of general wellness that go hand in hand with your nutritional efforts. You may enhance the benefits of the Blood Type Diet and promote your overall health and well-being by learning how to minimize stress and improve the quality of your sleep by adhering to these detailed instructions.

Step 1: Recognize the Effects of Sleep and Stress on Health

Start by realizing how stress and sleep are related to your general health. Acknowledge that several health problems, such as reduced immune function, elevated inflammation, weight gain, and mood disorders, can be attributed to long-term stress and poor sleep.

Recognize that, in addition to diet and exercise, stress management and good sleep hygiene are essential parts of your wellness regimen.

Step 2: Identify Sources of Stress

Take some time to identify sources of stress in your life, both external and internal. These may include work or school pressures, relationship conflicts, financial worries, health concerns, or personal insecurities.

Reflect on how these stressors impact your physical, mental, and emotional well-being, and consider strategies for addressing or mitigating them.

Step 3: Practice Stress-Reduction Techniques

Explore a variety of stress-reduction techniques to find what works best for you. This may include mindfulness meditation, deep breathing exercises, progressive muscle relaxation, yoga, tai chi, or guided imagery.

Incorporate stress-relief activities into your daily routine, such as taking short breaks to practice deep breathing, going for a walk in nature, or engaging in creative hobbies that bring you joy and relaxation.

Step 4: Cultivate Healthy Sleep Habits

Establish a consistent sleep schedule by going to bed and waking up at the same time each day, even on weekends. Aim for 7-9 hours of sleep per night, prioritizing quality over quantity.

Create a relaxing bedtime routine to signal to your body that it's time to wind down. This may include activities like taking a warm bath, reading a book, practicing gentle yoga or stretching, or listening to calming music or guided meditations.

Step 5: Create a Restful Sleep Environment

Set the stage for restful sleep by creating a comfortable and calming sleep environment. Keep your bedroom cool, dark, and quiet, and invest in a supportive mattress and pillows.

Limit exposure to screens (such as phones, computers, and TVs) before bedtime, as the blue light emitted can interfere with melatonin production and disrupt sleep patterns. Consider using blue light-blocking glasses or apps to minimize screen time in the evening.

Step 6: Limit Stimulants and Relax Before Bed

Avoid consuming stimulants like caffeine and nicotine close to bedtime, as they can interfere with your ability to fall asleep and stay asleep. Instead, opt for herbal teas or warm milk, which contain natural compounds that promote relaxation and sleep.

Engage in relaxing activities in the hour before bedtime to help calm your mind and prepare your body for sleep. This could include gentle stretching, meditation or mindfulness practices, journaling, or reading.

Step 7: Monitor and Adjust as Needed

Pay attention to your sleep patterns and stress levels over time, and be willing to make adjustments as needed to optimize your well-being.

Keep a sleep diary or use tracking apps to monitor your sleep habits and identify trends or patterns.

If you continue to struggle with stress or sleep despite your best efforts, consider seeking support from a healthcare professional or therapist who can provide additional guidance and resources.

By following these step-by-step guidelines for managing stress and improving sleep, you'll be better equipped to support your overall health and well-being alongside the dietary principles of the Blood Type Diet. In the final chapter, we'll recap key takeaways and offer encouragement as you continue on your journey toward optimal health and vitality.

CHAPTER 11

Summary and Next Steps

Welcome to the final chapter of your Blood Type Diet journey! In this chapter, we'll recap key takeaways from your exploration of the Blood Type Diet and offer guidance on the next steps as you continue on your path toward optimal health and vitality. By following these step-by-step guidelines, you've gained valuable insights into how to align your dietary choices with your unique blood type characteristics and support your overall well-being.

Step 1: Reflect on Your Journey

Take a moment to reflect on your journey through the Blood Type Diet. Consider the insights you've gained about your body's unique needs and preferences, as well as the changes you've made to your dietary habits and lifestyle.

Celebrate your successes and acknowledge any challenges you've faced along the way. Recognize the progress you've made toward improving your health and well-being, no matter how small.

Step 2: Recap Key Takeaways

Review the key principles and recommendations of the Blood Type Diet, tailored to your specific blood type (O, A, B, or AB). Recall the beneficial foods to include in your diet, as well as those to avoid or minimize.

Reflect on the strategies you've learned for meal planning and preparation, dining out, managing stress, improving sleep, and incorporating physical activity into your daily routine.

Step 3: Set Goals for Continued Progress

Set goals for continued progress on your wellness journey. Consider what areas of your health and lifestyle you'd like to focus on next, whether it's increasing physical activity, improving sleep quality, reducing stress, or refining your dietary choices.

Make your goals specific, measurable, achievable, relevant, and time-bound (SMART), and break them down into smaller, manageable steps to increase your chances of success.

Step 4: Stay Consistent and Flexible

Stay consistent with your dietary and lifestyle habits while remaining flexible and adaptable to change. Recognize that progress may not always be linear, and there will be ups and downs along the way.

Be patient with yourself and trust in the process of gradual, sustainable change. Focus on making small, incremental improvements over time, rather than striving for perfection.

Step 5: Seek Support and Accountability

Seek support from friends, family, or a health coach who can provide encouragement, accountability, and practical guidance on your journey. Share your goals and progress with others to stay motivated and accountable.

Consider joining online communities or support groups related to the Blood Type Diet, where you can connect with like-minded individuals and share experiences, tips, and recipes.

Step 6: Continue Learning and Growing

Stay curious and open to learning as you continue on your wellness journey. Explore new recipes, cooking techniques, and foods that align with your blood type and dietary preferences.

Stay informed about developments in nutrition science and research, and be willing to adjust your approach based on new information and insights.

Step 7: Celebrate Your Achievements

Finally, take time to celebrate your achievements and milestones along the way. Whether it's reaching a health goal, trying a new recipe, or incorporating a new self-care practice into your routine, acknowledge and celebrate your progress.

Remember that every step you take toward improving your health and well-being is a victory worth celebrating.

Congratulations on completing your journey through the Blood Type Diet! By following these step-by-step guidelines and incorporating the principles of the Blood Type Diet into your lifestyle, you've taken a proactive step toward optimizing your health and vitality. As you continue on your journey, may you find joy, fulfillment, and lasting well-being in nourishing your body and honoring its unique needs.

CHAPTER 12

FAQs and Troubleshooting

Welcome to Chapter 12, where we address common questions and concerns about the Blood Type Diet and provide troubleshooting tips for overcoming challenges along your journey. In this final chapter, we'll cover a range of topics to help you navigate

Step 1: Understanding Common Questions

any uncertainties and maintain confidence in your approach to the Blood Type Diet.

Begin by addressing frequently asked questions (FAQs) about the Blood Type Diet. These may include inquiries about the scientific basis of the diet, its effectiveness, and its potential benefits and limitations.

Provide clear and evidence-based answers to address common misconceptions and uncertainties, drawing upon the principles and recommendations outlined throughout the book.

Step 2: Clarifying Misunderstandings

Address any misunderstandings or misconceptions that may arise regarding the Blood Type Diet. This could involve debunking myths or misconceptions about specific blood types, food choices, or health outcomes associated with the diet.

Offer explanations supported by scientific evidence and encourage readers to approach the diet with an open mind while critically evaluating information.

Step 3: Troubleshooting Challenges

Identify common challenges or obstacles that individuals may encounter while following the Blood Type Diet. These could include difficulties with meal planning and preparation, dining out, managing cravings, or adhering to dietary recommendations.

Provide practical troubleshooting tips and strategies to overcome these challenges, such as simplifying meal plans, seeking support from friends or online communities, or experimenting with alternative ingredients or cooking methods.

Step 4: Addressing Individual Concerns

Acknowledge that each individual's experience with the Blood Type Diet may vary based on lifestyle, preferences, and health status. Encourage readers to listen to their bodies and adjust their approach as needed to suit their unique needs and circumstances.

Offer personalized guidance and support for addressing specific concerns or challenges raised by readers, whether related to weight management, energy levels, digestive issues, or other health considerations.

Step 5: Providing Additional Resources

Direct readers to additional resources for further information and support related to the Blood Type Diet. This could include reputable websites, books, research studies, or healthcare professionals specializing in integrative and functional medicine.

Empower readers to continue learning and exploring their health journey beyond the scope of this book, recognizing that ongoing education and self-discovery are integral to long-term success and well-being.

Step 6: Encouraging Persistence and Patience

Finally, encourage readers to persist in their journey toward better health and well-being, recognizing that meaningful change takes time and effort. Remind them that setbacks and challenges are normal and that small steps forward are still progress.

Offer words of encouragement and support, reminding readers of their resilience and capacity for growth as they continue to embrace the principles of the Blood Type Diet and prioritize their health.

By addressing frequently asked questions, clarifying misunderstandings, troubleshooting challenges, and providing additional resources and encouragement, this chapter aims to empower readers to navigate their blood-type diet journey with confidence and resilience. As you embark on this path toward optimal health and vitality, may you find fulfillment

and success in honoring your body's unique needs
and embracing a lifestyle that supports your
well-being.

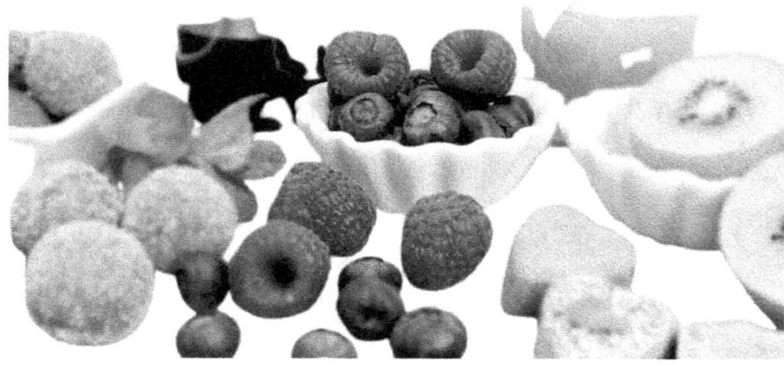

CHAPTER 13

Maintenance and Long-Term Success

Welcome to Chapter 13, where we'll explore strategies for maintaining your progress and achieving long-term success with the Blood Type Diet. In this final chapter, we'll provide step-by-step guidance on how to sustain your healthy habits, overcome obstacles, and continue thriving on your wellness journey for years to come.

Step 1: Reflect on Your Progress

Begin by reflecting on how far you've come since starting the Blood Type Diet. Celebrate your achievements, both big and small, and acknowledge the positive changes you've experienced in your health, energy levels, and overall well-being.

Take stock of the habits and strategies that have been most effective for you, as well as any areas where you may still have room for improvement.

Step 2: Establish Healthy Routines

Establish consistent routines that support your health and well-being every day. This may include regular meal times, dedicated time for exercise or physical activity, and bedtime rituals that promote restful sleep.

Incorporate self-care practices into your routine to nurture your mind, body, and spirit. This could involve mindfulness meditation, journaling, spending time in nature, or engaging in hobbies and activities that bring you joy.

Step 3: Monitor Your Progress

Continuously monitor your progress and track key indicators of health and wellness, such as weight, energy levels, mood, and physical fitness. Keep a journal or use digital tools to record your observations and track any changes over time.

Pay attention to how your body responds to different foods, activities, and lifestyle choices, and adjust your approach accordingly based on what works best for you.

Step 4: Stay Connected and Accountable

Stay connected with supportive friends, family members, or online communities that share your health and wellness goals. Share your successes, challenges, and progress with others, and seek encouragement and accountability when needed.

Consider partnering with an accountability buddy or joining a wellness group or program to stay motivated and on track with your goals.

Step 5: Adaptability and Flexibility

Remain flexible and adaptable in your approach to health and wellness. Recognize that life is full of changes and unexpected challenges, and be willing to adjust your routines and strategies as needed to navigate these transitions.

Embrace a growth mindset and view setbacks or obstacles as opportunities for learning and growth. Approach challenges with resilience and a willingness to problem-solve and explore new solutions.

Step 6: Celebrate Milestones and Successes

Celebrate milestones and successes along your journey, no matter how small they may seem. Whether it's reaching a weight loss goal, completing a fitness challenge, or mastering a new healthy recipe, take time to acknowledge and celebrate your achievements.

Cultivate a sense of gratitude for the progress you've made and the positive changes you've experienced in your health and well-being.

Step 7: Embrace Lifelong Learning and Growth

Finally, embrace the journey of lifelong learning and growth as you continue on your path toward optimal health and vitality. Stay curious, open-minded, and receptive to new information, insights, and opportunities for self-improvement.

Commit to investing in your health and well-being as a lifelong priority, recognizing that small, consistent efforts over time can lead to profound and lasting transformation.

By following these step-by-step guidelines for maintenance and long-term success with the Blood Type Diet, you'll be better equipped to sustain your progress and continue thriving on your wellness journey for years to come. As you embrace a lifestyle that supports your unique needs and honors your body's wisdom, may you experience continued health, vitality, and fulfillment in all aspects of your life?

CHAPTER 14

Beyond the Blood Type Diet: Integrating Holistic Wellness

Welcome to Chapter 14, where we'll explore the broader concept of holistic wellness beyond the confines of the Blood Type Diet. In this final chapter, we'll provide step-by-step guidance on how to integrate various aspects of holistic health into your lifestyle, encompassing physical, mental, emotional, and spiritual well-being.

Step 1: Embracing Holistic Wellness

Begin by embracing the concept of holistic wellness, which recognizes the interconnectedness of mind, body, and spirit in achieving optimal health and vitality. Understand that true wellness encompasses more than just dietary choices and extends to all areas of life.

Shift your perspective to view health as a dynamic and multifaceted journey that involves nourishing your body, nurturing your relationships, cultivating a positive mindset, and aligning with your values and purpose.

Step 2: Nourishing Your Body

Continue to prioritize nourishing your body with nutrient-dense foods that support your health and well-being. Build upon the principles of the Blood Type Diet by incorporating a diverse array of whole foods, including fruits, vegetables, lean proteins, healthy fats, and whole grains.

Explore other dietary approaches, such as plant-based or Mediterranean-inspired eating patterns, that align with your preferences and nutritional needs. Focus on food quality, mindful eating, and intuitive eating practices to foster a positive relationship with food.

Step 3: Cultivating Physical Health

Cultivate physical health and vitality through regular exercise, movement, and physical activity. Incorporate a variety of activities that you enjoy, including cardiovascular exercise, strength training, flexibility exercises, and outdoor recreation.

Prioritize movement throughout your day by integrating short bursts of activity, taking active breaks, and incorporating movement into daily tasks and routines. Listen to your body and honor its need for rest, recovery, and rejuvenation.

Step 4: Nurturing Mental and Emotional Well-Being

Nurture your mental and emotional well-being through practices that promote stress reduction, relaxation, and emotional resilience. Explore mindfulness meditation, deep breathing exercises, yoga, tai chi, or other mind-body practices that resonate with you.

Cultivate self-awareness and emotional intelligence by practicing self-reflection, journaling, and mindfulness. Prioritize self-care activities that replenish your energy and uplift your spirits, such as spending time in nature, connecting with loved ones, or engaging in creative pursuits.

Step 5: Fostering Social Connections

Foster meaningful social connections and relationships that nourish your soul and provide support and companionship along your wellness journey. Invest time and energy in nurturing friendships, family bonds, and community connections.

Seek out opportunities for meaningful engagement and contribution, whether through volunteering, participating in group activities or hobbies, or joining clubs or organizations that align with your interests and values.

Step 6: Cultivating Spiritual Well-Being

Cultivate spiritual well-being by exploring practices that foster a sense of connection, purpose, and meaning in your life. This may involve engaging in spiritual or religious practices, connecting with nature, or exploring mindfulness and meditation.

Reflect on your values, beliefs, and sense of purpose, and identify ways to align your actions with your deepest aspirations and intentions. Cultivate gratitude, compassion, and forgiveness as pathways to spiritual growth and fulfillment.

Step 7: Embracing Lifelong Growth and Evolution

Embrace the journey of lifelong growth and evolution as you continue to explore and integrate holistic wellness practices into your life. Stay curious, open-minded, and receptive to new experiences, insights, and opportunities for learning and growth.

Recognize that wellness is a dynamic and evolving process that requires ongoing attention, intention, and commitment. Trust in your innate capacity for healing and transformation, and embrace each moment as an opportunity to thrive and flourish.

By embracing the principles of holistic wellness and integrating them into your lifestyle, you'll cultivate a foundation of health, vitality, and fulfillment that extends far beyond the confines of any specific diet or regimen. As you continue on your journey of self-discovery and well-being, may you find joy, abundance, and meaning in every aspect of your life.

Conclusion:

Your Journey to Vibrant Health and Wellness

Welcome to the final chapter of your journey toward vibrant health and wellness. In this concluding chapter, we'll reflect on the transformative journey you've undertaken and offer guidance as you embark on the next phase of your wellness evolution. Let's explore the key insights and steps you've taken to nurture your body, mind, and spirit, and celebrate the progress you've made along the way.

Step 1: Reflecting on Your Journey

Take a moment to reflect on the journey you've undertaken throughout this book. Recall the insights you've gained, the challenges you've overcome, and the growth you've experienced along the way.

Celebrate your commitment to prioritizing your health and well-being, and acknowledge the positive changes you've made in your dietary habits, lifestyle choices, and mindset.

Step 2: Recognizing Your Achievements

Recognize and celebrate your achievements, no matter how small they may seem. Whether you've made strides in adopting healthier eating habits, incorporating regular exercise into your routine, or cultivating a more positive outlook on life, every step forward is a victory worth celebrating.

Acknowledge the progress you've made toward becoming the healthiest and happiest version of yourself, and give yourself credit for the dedication and effort you've invested in your wellness journey.

Step 3: Embracing Your Unique Path

Embrace the uniqueness of your wellness journey and honor the path that's unfolded for you. Recognize that there's no one-size-fits-all approach to health and well-being and that what works for others may not necessarily be the best fit for you.

Trust in your body's innate wisdom and intuition, and continue to listen to its signals and cues as you navigate your path toward optimal health and vitality.

Step 4: Cultivating Gratitude and Appreciation

Cultivate a sense of gratitude and appreciation for the journey you've embarked on and the lessons you've learned along the way. Be grateful for the abundance of nourishing foods that support your health, the opportunities for movement and physical activity that invigorate your body, and the relationships and connections that enrich your life.

Practice gratitude daily by reflecting on the blessings and gifts in your life, no matter how small, and expressing appreciation for the abundance that surrounds you.

Step 5: Setting Intentions for the Future

Set intentions for the future based on your aspirations and desires for continued growth and evolution. Consider what areas of your health and well-being you'd like to focus on next, and set specific goals that align with your values and priorities.

Make your intentions clear and actionable, and create a plan of action to support their realization. Break down your goals into manageable steps and milestones, and commit to taking consistent, intentional action toward their achievement.

Step 6: Embracing Lifelong Learning and Growth

Embrace the journey of lifelong learning and growth as you continue to evolve on your path toward vibrant health and wellness. Stay curious, open-minded, and receptive to new ideas, experiences, and opportunities for personal and spiritual development.

Cultivate a growth mindset that views challenges as opportunities for learning and transformation, and approach each day with a sense of curiosity, wonder, and possibility.

Step 7: Trusting in Your Inner Wisdom

Trust in your inner wisdom and intuition as you navigate your wellness journey. Tune into the signals and messages your body, mind, and spirit send you, and honor your intuition as a guide for making decisions that align with your highest good.

Remember that you are the expert in your own body and life, and trust that you have the wisdom and resources within you to create the vibrant, fulfilling life you desire.

As you conclude this book and embark on the next phase of your wellness journey, may you continue to prioritize your health, happiness, and vitality, and may you find joy, fulfillment, and abundance in every moment. Remember that your journey toward vibrant health and wellness is ongoing and that every step you take brings you closer to embodying the vibrant, radiant being you were meant to be.